HOW TO DRIVE HIM CRAZY IN BED

The Ultimate Guide to Seducing, Tease, and Riding Your Man in Bed

Paul D. Wold

Table of content

Chapter 1

The technique of sexual teasing is the perfect way to liven up your relationship with your partner in the bedroom. It's a lighthearted and seductive approach to ratcheting things up and setting the stage for a passionate evening for the two of you. However, how precisely does one tease a man sexually? These are our best strategies and pointers to help you become an expert in sexual teasing.

A Beginner's Guide to Understanding the Art of Sexual Teasing

Let's examine what sexual teasing is in more detail before getting into the details. Building sexual tension and a sense of anticipation for what's to come are the fundamental goals of sexual teasing. It's a method to spark your partner's creativity and leave him wanting more. Sexual taunting may range from lighthearted conversation to physical contact and all in between.

It's crucial to remember that polite and consenting sexual taunting is always appropriate. It's not about controlling or coercing your significant other into doing anything against their will. Rather, it's about discovering fresh avenues for personal connection and jointly exploring your wants. When it comes to sexual teasing, communication is essential, so be sure that both of you are okay with the amount of teasing you're exchanging.

Why It's Okay to Make Sexual Jokes in Your Relationship

In addition to being a flirtatious and enjoyable method to liven up your bedroom scene, sexual teasing may also be beneficial to your relationship overall. You're developing closeness and trust in your relationship with your boyfriend by teasing him sexually. Additionally, it can aid in preventing the regularity and monotony that occasionally seeps into committed partnerships.

Additionally, it has been shown that sexual teasing improves understanding and communication between couples. It makes it possible to have frank discussions about boundaries and wants, which may result in a more rewarding and happy sexual encounter for both people. Furthermore, because it produces endorphins and generates a feeling of excitement and anticipation, sexual teasing can aid in stress reduction and relaxation.

Mood-Setting: Establishing the Ideal Scene for Sexual Joking

The correct setting is essential for successful sexual teasing. Make sure you create the right atmosphere with cozy furnishings, sensual music, and gentle lighting. For your man to participate completely in the experience, you want him to feel at ease and at ease. To further elevate the atmosphere, think about adding silk bedding or indulging in some sensuous aromatherapy.

Anticipation has a significant role in establishing the tone for sexual tease. Build up the sexual tension gradually by starting with playful touches or murmurs that tease your lover. You both will have a more thrilling and pleasurable encounter as a result.

Lastly, remember to be in constant communication with your partner during the event. Inquire about their preferences and desires, and be receptive to their input. By doing this, you can better cater the experience to their preferences and guarantee a fun time for the two of you.

How to Look Good: Selecting the Appropriate Clothing for Sexual Joking

What you dress matters when it comes to sexual teasing just as much as the atmosphere you create. Pick an ensemble that exudes confidence and sexiness while leaving room for interpretation. A silky robe, a form-fitting dress, or lingerie are all excellent choices. You want to arouse curiosity in your partner about what lies beneath.

When selecting your attire for sexual teasing, it's crucial to take the occasion and environment into account as well. More revealing clothing can be suitable if you're planning a night in. But if you're heading out in public, remember that not every situation calls for a certain article of clothing. Always exercise your best judgment and take into account other people's possible reactions.

How to Seduce Someone with Your Eyes: The Power of Eye Contact

Making eye contact with a man is an effective way to tease him sexually. Make eye contact with your partner and maintain eye contact while flashing a seductive grin or teasing wink. Making eye contact may enhance intimacy and foster a stronger connection, which can enhance your enjoyment of the event together.

But it's crucial to keep in mind that there are other ways to entice your lover than making eye contact. Try a variety of approaches, including whispering in his ear or giving him a seductive touch. Intimacy and increased sexual tension can also be produced by these behaviors.

It's also critical to confirm that your spouse feels at ease with the amount of eye contact and playful sexual taunting. In every sexual experience, communication is essential, so be sure to check in with your partner and inquire about their preferences and boundaries.

Techniques for Flirting That Will
Make Him Crazy

A crucial element of sexual teasing
is flirting. To spark your man's
curiosity, engage in lighthearted
conversation and provocative
comments. To further improve the
experience, try adding some subtle
touches or amusing movements.

Keeping eye contact is another
useful flirtatious tactic. Making
eye contact with your partner may
strengthen your bond and
heighten the climactic moments.
Moreover, make an effort to
mimic his gestures and body

language to foster mutual understanding and a sense of togetherness between you both. Always remember to make things lighthearted and fun, and don't be scared to try new things and take chances!

Touches That Feel Real and Will Make Him Want More

Physical contact still plays a significant role in the experience even if the main goal of sexual teasing is to create anticipation. To further arouse your partner and leave him wanting more, think about adding soft touches or tender caresses. Just remember to respect his boundaries and pay attention to his indications.

It's crucial to remember that everyone has distinct preferences for physical contact. While some people might prefer a gentler touch, others could appreciate a tight grasp or rough play. Understanding your partner's interests and comfort zones requires open communication. Ask for input when you need it, and don't be hesitant to modify your strategy. Recall that the objective is to improve the experience for both parties.

Using Dirty Talk to Make Sexual Teasing More Enjoyable

One of the best ways to improve the sensation of sexual teasing is with dirty words. Employ innuendos and provocative words to pique your man's interest in what could be coming. When you introduce foul language into your routine of sexual teasing, be sure to understand his signs and respect his boundaries.

It's critical to keep in mind that not everyone enjoys nasty comments. It could make some individuals uneasy or even angered. Have an honest discussion about your partner's comfort level and boundaries before using sexual teasing tactics such as dirty language.

It's also critical to remember that unpleasant conversations should never be exchanged against consent. It's crucial to pause and check in with your partner if they don't appear comfortable or are not responding favorably. In any sexual encounter, communication

is essential, and nasty
conversation is no different.

Playing Role-Playing Games Can
Be Fun and Exciting

Consider adding some
role-playing games to your routine
of sexual tease if you're feeling
daring. To make the encounter
more exciting and original, dress
up in costume or act out certain
events.

Couples can explore their
imaginations and wants in a
consenting and safe manner by
engaging in role-playing games.
Partners can experiment with

power dynamics and attempt new things that they would not feel comfortable doing in their daily lives by assuming various roles.

Setting up limits and communicating openly is crucial before playing any role-playing games. Make sure there is a safe phrase in place in case things become too heated and that both parties are at ease with the situation. Recall that the objective is to enjoy yourself and your intercourse, not to cause discomfort or fear to others.

Tips for Maintaining Consensus During Sexual Joking

When engaging in sexual teasing, it's critical to always put consent and respect first. Make sure you and your partner have excellent communication and pay close attention to his limits and indications. Before taking on any new tasks or situations, go slowly and develop a secure and transparent communication channel.

Making frequent check-ins with your spouse is another crucial component of maintaining a consenting relationship during sexual teasing. Find out from them how they are feeling and whether they are at ease with the situation. Make sure to pause and address their concerns before moving on if they show any signs of discomfort or doubt.

Furthermore, it's critical to keep in mind that consent is a continuous process rather than a one-time commitment. Continue to check in with your partner to see if they're still comfortable and eager to join as you explore new scenarios or activities. Additionally, always honor their requests and put their well-being first if they ever express a want to stop or take a break.

The Advantages of Using Sexual Teasing to Push Your Relationship's Boundaries

It may be thrilling and satisfying for you and your partner to push limits and attempt new things. A wonderful method to test your limits and discover new possibilities in your relationship is to tease each other sexually. Just remember to put respect and communication first before attempting anything new.

The promotion of closeness and trust between lovers is one advantage of sexual teasing. A stronger connection and mutual understanding of wants and desires can arise when both of you feel confident enough to attempt new things and explore new limits.

The ability to maintain the spark in your relationship is yet another advantage of sexual teasing. Pushing limits and doing new things may keep things interesting and prevent the relationship from getting monotonous or stale. Additionally, it might provide you both a stronger sense of self-worth and sexual empowerment.

Advice on How to Effectively Express Your Boundaries and Desires During Sexual Teasing

It takes open and honest communication between you and your guy to pull off a successful sexual tease. Make sure you are clear about your expectations and boundaries, and pay close attention to his wants and worries as well. Your experience will be better the more you communicate.

Setting limits before engaging in sexual taunting is crucial. This might involve talking about what is and isn't acceptable behavior as well as what phrases or behaviors can cause pain or distress. Throughout the teasing, it's crucial to periodically check in with each other to make sure that everyone is at ease and having fun.

Recall that dialogue is a two-way process. Encourage your spouse to express their limits and desires as well. You both may have a more equitable and satisfying encounter as a result of this. To make sure you are both on the same page during the tease, don't be scared to clarify anything or offer criticism.

The Value of Mutual Respect and Trust in Sexual Teasing

Any effective sexual teasing technique must include both trust and respect. Always put your partner's needs and limits first, and make sure the space is secure and welcoming so that you may both enjoy the experience to the fullest. You may advance your sexual teasing routine by establishing mutual respect and trust.

When it comes to sexual teasing, it's critical to be transparent and honest with your partner about your preferences and boundaries.

This can guarantee that there is a foundation of mutual respect and trust and that both partners feel secure and at ease throughout the encounter. Always pay attention to your partner's input and modify your strategy as necessary to build a stronger relationship based on mutual respect and trust.

Typical Errors to Avoid When Making Sexual Jokes About a Man

There are a few typical blunders that can ruin the whole experience of sexually teasing a man. These flaws might stop the flow of the conversation. Always pay attention to your partner's indications to make sure he's comfortable with the situation and refrain from being overly forceful or aggressive. Never be scared to start slowly and increase the intensity bit by bit. Throughout the entire process, put communication and respect first.

You'll be well on your way to being an expert at sexual teasing and improving your relationship if you adhere to these pointers and strategies. Consent, respect, and communication should always come first. Enjoy pushing the envelope and trying new things with your partner.

When making sexual jokes about a man, it's also typical to make the error of concentrating just on physical contact. In addition to verbal teasing and building a mental bond with your partner, touch is a crucial component in sexual teasing. Don't be scared to explore many imaginations and scenarios with your partner; use your words to generate excitement and develop anticipation.

Finally, it's critical to keep in mind that sexual teasing ought to be a pleasurable and consenting activity for both parties involved. Respecting your partner's limits and being honest about your feelings is crucial if they ever show discomfort or ask you to stop. You and your partner may have a satisfying and thrilling sexual encounter if you put mutual enjoyment, respect, and communication first.

chapter 2

Seducing your lover may be like the first rain in the sweltering summer months, whether you are just starting and want to heat things or you are in a committed relationship and want to add some zing. Following is a great deal of satisfaction, pleasure, and expectation. And we lay out for you the precise steps to woo a man.

"Seduction does not force someone to do something against

their will. Someone is being lured into doing what they have been wanting to accomplish all along. Whoever stated the words above perfectly captured the essence of seduction. Some refer to seduction as witchcraft, yet we completely agree that it is an art form, similar to pottery or building.

Some describe seduction as "a game of psychology, not beauty," adding that "anyone can become a master at the game." It's accurate. A game of excitement, desire, discovery, and satiation is seduction. It's a necessary talent to spice up your connection in the romantic world.

In a protracted and boring relationship, sometimes seduction is what brings life back to life when things go dry. Everybody will have to play the seducer at some time in their life. Thus, you have to familiarize yourself with the guidelines right away. On the brighter side, wooing your mate is a lot of fun. Here are some methods for you and your partner to enjoy the journey and master the art of seduction.

How To Entice Your Partner And Make Him Want More

You are mistaken if you believe that seduction only made the evening more interesting. Your relationship with your lover is strengthened and elevated by the art of seduction, where you both become each other's dream come true. You only need to have a little kinkiness and the purpose to entice your lover to start having hot and steamy relationships.

You may strengthen your connection and reignite the flame in your relationship when you make a man hunger for you. You'll have him pleading for more of you in no time. Your partner must have envisaged you making that sensual walk in a golden bikini someday, even if he would not confess it.

Everyone enjoys being seduced, although not many people may admit it outright. Thus, you may be certain that your significant other is only anticipating your next move. Similarly, even though you may want to blow your man's mind, it's possible that your inhibitions get the better of you and you are at a loss for words. But what if you could woo your significant other without speaking? You did read correctly.

There exist several methods to physically entice a man without resorting to derogatory speech. Interested? With these 18 foolproof suggestions, let's get this tutorial on how to entice a man underway:

1. Mock him

This is a tried-and-true method that is easy to use to entice a man without saying anything. Wear lacy, see-through pajamas, and be nude below. As you tease him, keep your distance from him. You might also try eating chocolate that has melted and licking your fingers while glaring at him now and again.

2. Adopt the no-hands policy.

Maybe the simplest method to make a man want you more than ever is to let him stare at you but not touch you. Should your ruse succeed, he will crave more. Tell him, however, that using his hands is not permitted. That will arouse him even more. You'll observe the inventiveness with which males may come up with ideas.

3. A filthy text

With the ease of access to technology, there are several methods to entice your partner even when they are not in physical proximity. Use messages to flirt with your boyfriend when he's at work or elsewhere. It will instill in him a sense of expectation. mention something along the lines of "I want to do things with you today that are so wild I can't say them." He would probably be seeking reasons to get home and show you a nice time.

Send him a filthy text.

4. Send captivating images

You have to make an effort if you want to physically seduce a man. What better way to do it than with a sophisticated yet alluring photo? No, we're not talking about nudity; rather, we're talking about something like a transparent, braless top. or a short skirt that only shows off your buttocks' shape. This is the type of image that will cause his hormones to wake up. Soon, expect him home.

5. Go shopping with him

Not your typical trip to the mall, that is. That's one method to entice your boyfriend, as you and we both know. It will, if anything, destroy his libido. We are discussing shopping for underwear. If all you want to say to a man is, "We're going lingerie shopping and you get to pick," then this is going to work. Get him to sit close to the trial room so he can have a look. Is he willing to take them from you right then and there? Of course, You can woo your boyfriend by doing this.

6. Catch him off guard with a sexy glance

Long-term relationships don't give a damn about your appearance.

Your dress code is pajamas and a disheveled bun. However, when he rings the doorbell the following time, welcome him with your hair parted, wear little makeup, and be yourself as normal. He will become inquisitively aroused. That's how you talk no words at all and seduce a man. This concludes your role as a seductress. Now is the moment to move things forward.

7. After that, undress.

When his inquisitiveness starts to overwhelm him, force him to sit on the couch, offer him a drink, and take off your underwear and bra in front of him. It's much better if you pretend to be a fool. He'll follow you around with his mouth agape, just like a good puppy would. This is an amazing method to entice a man. Just for you, a few more bedroom secrets!

An amazing method to entice a male

8. Make love, then turn away

How do you entice a man and make him go insane? by satiating his desire for more? Give him whatever he wants, then leave before the last act to take a shower or make up an excuse about having to attend an all-night party. Observe his desire for you while he lies in bed. But please, don't be a tease; return and complete the task at hand.

9. Join him for a shower

Enter the restroom covertly with him while he's not expecting it. A man is best approached physically in the shower, especially when he isn't expecting it. It will arouse the two of you. Play around with him, maybe even engage in some foreplay, and advise him to keep that idea in his head for the remainder of the day. When you two come together at the end of the day, we guarantee the finest sex of your life.

10. Take off your perfume

Apply your preferred fragrance or scented hairspray. Stroll, spreading your enticing aroma all about him. He would, well, go insane. Use the science that exists between scent and emotion to your benefit. If you're searching for nonverbal methods to entice a man, a hint of the perfect scent is the way to go.

11. Set the tone

A simple romantic gesture is one of the most effective methods to entice a man. Adopt a traditional strategy and give it your best. You wait for him with roses as you light fragrant candles, play live music, and wear a skimpy one-piece. Though it may appear laborious, we assure you that it is worthwhile. It's worthwhile to woo a man.

12. Act as his masseur.

Ways to entice a man? by allowing him to enjoy your contact without understanding the consequences. Make sure to contact his erogenous zones throughout the massage. A bite through his earlobes, a kiss on his throat, a circle around his navel rings. You touch him, and his body will react in ways you can never predict. Even try your hand at filthy dancing.

17. Try a different sleeping posture

When women take the lead in bed, guys like it. So give him a mind-blowing performance of daring new maneuvers on the bed. He will undoubtedly return to you for more. Seek advice from your friends, educate yourself on sex roles, or search for his favorite porn online and take cues from it. You'll blow his mind if you try this, girl.

18. Acquire some sensual skills

The appropriate dancing moves will capture him in minutes if they are done correctly. You may pick out some attractive clothes after learning a few movements. You may play peek-a-boo or striptease while dancing, always revealing some of your body while concealing others. Are you aware of men's erogenous zones? If not, you ought to make an effort to solve them.

These 18 techniques can help you win over your man's body and mind, ladies. Turning him on isn't always the goal of the art of seduction. It's a fun and highly helpful way to make your relationship stronger with your partner. But always remember the golden rule: you shouldn't give him everything at once. The goal is always to leave him wanting more. Start plotting and organizing now. He's got time!

chapter 3

If you've never done it in bed, one of his hottest dreams is to be ridden by a lady, and he's yearning to do it. Standing, side by side, or even as a missionary, there is nothing like the penetrating sense of riding a guy. Given that you are usually the one causing the friction, even the orgasm feels different.

Riding a man till he shows up and begs you to continue, then stop, then start going again, then stop, is a bit of an acquired technique. Being in charge of his orgasm and having complete control over it is a beautiful, enthusiastic experience.

Initially, it won't seem as effortless as it will eventually. You could feel uncomfortable and wonder simple things like, "Should I jump up and down?" or "Should I rock back and forth slowly?"

Tips for Riding your man

Today, we'll address all of your riding inquiries on how to ride a guy. And you'll be able to quip, half-jokingly, that this isn't your first rodeo by the conclusion of the book!

Try a variety of postures first.

It's quite kinky to sit on top of his lap, especially if you mix it with a lap dance. Both the "woman-on-top" and "reverse cowgirl" poses are excellent choices for photos. If you truly want to make his head spin, switch things up and keep him wondering.

2. Take note of the penis!

Naturally, a "broken penis" is the worst-case scenario, but it is not unheard of. Many men suffer injuries from, uh, "riding accidents." It is therefore preferable to observe his penis and how deep within he is. If you want to ride him hard for a few minutes, be cautious not to let him fall out. Before you fully rest your weight on him, especially if you're both seated, make sure he's comfortable. The greatest method to prevent damage is to match him at your "natural angle" together.

While bouncing, grinding, and rolling are enjoyable, the slower, "fuller" in-and-out stroke is the most effective in providing him with pleasure and safeguarding his penis. It makes sure you don't fall at an odd angle unexpectedly

and stimulates his shaft and penis
head.

3. You can sway, grind, hop, or
roll. The choice is yours.

When it comes to riding him at a
certain velocity, there is no correct
answer. Everything feels nice, but
when you're just starting, it's best
to rock or sway more slowly. As
your desire grows together, you
may try a more forceful grinding
motion or perhaps a "rolling"
motion with your butt and hips.
The greatest danger of harm
comes from jumping, which is also
what you frequently see in
pornographic images. Before you

descend after that huge splash, it's crucial that you genuinely monitor his penis to make sure he's not falling out. Another option is to do a slower variation of the leap, such as an up-and-down pull-up and stroke, which is deliberate enough to guarantee he's always inside of you upon landing.

4. Bend forward to give him complete control over your body.

Don't deny him dessert since "boobs in the face" is one of the finest benefits of being a woman on top. Just slightly bend down so he can get to you. His want is for the fondling, not simply the visual thrill. Hugs, kisses, and even cheek-to-cheek contact make the experience better.

5. Steady does it; he does not constantly shift places.

Changing positions might perhaps be beneficial if you're trying to avoid ejaculating too soon. The secret is to establish a steady, continuous rhythm and keep repeating it for as long as he can tolerate it if you're ready for him to have an orgasm. Of course, you shouldn't try bouncing or jumping if you lack the necessary stamina. Instead, pick a rolling motion that you can easily perform for a few minutes at a time.

6. Unwind and assume command.

To start, when a woman assumes leadership, males adore it! Thus, this fantastic role! It's time to unwind and have fun now that you know that. He wants you to ride him in part so you can force yourself to come. He wants you to follow your instincts since, more often than not, they will serve him well as well! When determining the ideal spot position, angle, and MOTION, take your time. Determine which rhythm and angle activate your G-spot the most. The amount of noise he is making makes it easy to determine how much he is loving it!

Furthermore, you can be sure that he would prefer you to orgasm first and then return to finish him off rather than worrying about you orgasming first and him orgasming first. Because of the potential for extreme visual and auditory stimulation, he could be so turned on that he orgasms when you do. Which gets us to the next point.

7. While you're riding, touch yourself or allow him to touch you.

Climatic stimulation will be beneficial regardless of whether you can locate your G-spot in this posture. In addition to providing manual clitoral stimulation, woman-on-top enables you to feel vaginal penetration (maybe even G-spot, as straddling permits entry at an angle). Allow him to touch you while you are riding him, or touch yourself instead. It will only intensify and enhance your riding experience together.

8. Maintain close eye contact throughout the whole journey.

This is where tantric love is at! Making intense eye contact while riding intensifies the experience and strengthens the emotional connection. As he ogles your breasts, remind him how amazing riding can be by forcing him to look directly into your eyes while you straddle him for an orgasm.

9. Rub all over him.

Concentrating while riding, defending him, and getting off yourself is difficult. But if you take the time to touch him, he'll give you an additional sigh of gratitude. Caressing his face, reaching for his stomach or chest, or gently rubbing his testicles can all intensify the impending complete-body orgasm.

10. Lastly, exude confidence!

I understand that it will be difficult for you to let go of your inhibitions and embrace your inner sex vixen, but you need to take control of this moment. You need to be certain that he wants you and that by giving in to all of his desires, you would cause him to lose it. Discuss his desires with him before, after, and during so that you are on the same page.

on the same page. He'll feel the same way if you're feeling free and happy. It's positive energy that you desire!

Enjoy yourself while playing with this novel approach to making love, and keep trying until you've tried a few different "riding" styles. Not only can practicing help one become flawless, but it's also a lot of fun!

There are several methods you may use to elicit a man's groan in bed. Here's a comprehensive instruction on making a man groan in bed if he wants to make things so heated during sex that he sheds tears of ecstasy.

Scream his name a lot.

Ironically, a man's name is among the many things he enjoys hearing during sex. When you enjoy something sexual that he's doing to you, call out his name in a seductive manner. Oh, please keep the name of the person you are sleeping with exactly in mind. Before uttering someone else's name.

Speak with him.

Hearing each other sigh, complain, and demand what you want, how you want it, is the epitome of sex. It assures you both of the same level of enjoyment. Furthermore, speaking inappropriate things in his ears might be quite enticing. Use this information any way you see fit.

Make fun of his ears.

Playfully bite it or just give it a little tug. You might even simply sigh or groan in his ears. You should do this if you want the sex to stick in his memory since the ears can be an erogenous zone.

Pay close attention to his neck

To let him know you desire him, start with soft kisses. Work your way down from the base of his ears. You may gently bite down on his neck, inch by inch. Switch up your kissing and biting so he never knows what to expect next.

Search for his weak points.

You have to deliberately try to please a man sexually if you want to know how to make him cry in bed.

Men have a lot of erogenous zones that go unloved, primarily because they are too hesitant to approach their spouses to request it. One of those places is the breasts. Be mindful of it. Simply do to you what he would do.

Curl up his thighs.

Start lightly kissing him above his legs and gradually raise your lips pressure as you advance. Recall that males like foreplay as well.

Give a massage to him.

Place your mouth and tongue in place of your hands as you massage him while straddling him. He should find this to be an intriguing experience.

Try adjusting the temperature.

Introduce novel items into the bedroom, such as whipped cream, ice, and skin-care candles.

Unwind

Not everything will go as planned. Sex can't be flawless between two individuals who aren't performing to get money. Let loose, chuckle,

and crack jokes. Enjoy yourselves,
please.